PHYSICIAN FREEDOM

Living Your Authentic Physician Life

Dispel career confusion, streamline
decision making, and be true to your
vision and values

DR. FRANCIS YOO, D.O.

DISCLAIMER: The information provided in this book is designed to provide information and motivation and is not meant to be used, nor should it be used, to diagnose or treat any medical condition. The author and publisher are not responsible for any specific health needs that may require medical supervision and are not liable for any damages or negative consequences from any action to any person reading or following the information in this book. Or, in other words, this book is meant to give you a framework and method for introspection and self-discovery, and you are responsible for whatever it is that you discover and what actions you take afterward. Readers should be aware that the websites listed in this book may change.

CONTENTS

FRANCIS YOO

###

Introduction

Is this book for you?

Hey there! Thanks for picking up this book. As the title suggests, I wrote this book for physicians and physicians-to-be who are experiencing the sensations of "being stuck," restricted, blocked, lost, disconnected, or unfulfilled in relation to their being a physician. If any of these describe you, keep on reading! If not, consider recommending it to someone who comes to mind.

Still here?

Good!

Now, I do not know your situation or the level of urgency you have to try and improve your situation, but before you rush out to get a new job, start your own private practice, embark on a non-clinical career, climb Mt. Kilimanjaro in less than 36 hours with Wim

Hof, or whatever you think will make your life better - read this book and use it to help figure out where it is that you want to go.

Before we get started, you have to know that this book will require you to engage in introspection and inner work. There are two ways to read this book: 1) Take your time to do each exercise when presented, or 2) Read through the whole thing in one sitting, then re-read while doing the exercises in depth at a slower pace. Either one will work. It's all about what works best for you right now.

Also, dig out the personal statement that you wrote for either your medical school and/or residency application. You will need it for Chapter 1.

Your "well-being"

You have probably noticed that physician well-being is a hot topic, not only in medical news and literature, but increasingly in non-medical media as well. Terms such as burnout, moral injury, dissatisfaction, suicide are increasingly being associated with physicians in the United States and internationally. One important reason for this is the discombobulation of the medical world we inhabit.

Discombobulation

It is not a secret that both the United States healthcare system and associated medical culture are quite discombobulated. And this system is really at odds with the reason you became a physician in the first place. Many physicians are practicing medicine in a system and culture that does not prioritize patient care and is unsupportive of their values, time, goals.

For example, in one of the outpatient primary care centers I have worked at, giving the patient their "patient plan" was one of the metrics that was measured. However, generating a patient plan document and giving it to the patient was not a data point captured by the system. I had to go to a separate tab and click the box next to the "patient plan" just to get the system to recognize that I had done this. Nod your head if you can feel my pain.

Part of this discombobulation, in fact a key component, is that many aspects of corporate medicine, including school and residency, are built to make you replaceable. (Check out Seth Godin's material on "Stop stealing dreams (What is school for?)" https://seths.blog/2014/09/the-shameful-fraud-of-sorting-for-youth-meritocracy/

To illustrate, try this thought experiment: let's say you die while being an employed physician. Which is posted first: your obituary or a job posting to replace you?

How to fix this?

If you go and sort through the many, many proposed solutions in the blogs, medical journals, practice management journals, etc., you will see that there are generally three strategies:

Change the system or culture for the better.

Give you resources so that you can perform your work better.

Give you resources to change your work situation.

Let's briefly look at each one.

Changing the system or culture for the better

Imagine a health care system that prioritizes and fully supports the health and well-being of patients and their physicians. Moreover, one where the government, hospital systems, residency programs, medical schools, clinics, and health care teams' cultures all function to do the same. This would GREAT!

But obviously far, far from reality.

Now it would be great if changes that lead to this improved system and culture could happen, but it is going to take a lot of work. And how long would it take? Can you afford to wait? If not, can you afford to try and change the system on your own? To you, this may seem like one more overbearing item that is added to your to-do list.

Resources to perform current work better

Examples include:

- ➤ Alleviating documentation load by providing a scribe or dictation option
- ➤ Redesigning workflow with Lean Six Sigma or other methodologies
- ➤ Providing events that are supposed to promote self-care (massage, yoga, meditation)

These all sound nice. However it is important to note that the main goal of this strategy is to keep the physician in their current role (workforce retention); that is, the employer has interests *past* simply making sure you are doing well – they simply want to keep you around.

Resources to change the work situation

Examples include:

➢ Helping physicians start and run cash-only private practices

➢ Helping physicians gain new skills (procedure workshops and courses)

➢ Non-clinical career options, including coaching for career transitions

This is the most physician-focused approach and is a growing market. Do a search for "physician career change coach," and you will get PLENTY of results.

Your development

Now each of these strategies have their place and can be beneficial for you, and I am in no way diminishing their usefulness (I am a Lean Six Sigma green belt and have benefited greatly from it).

The problem is that their focus is not on the MOST crucial aspect:

YOU.

You are an individual with your circumstances, your environment, your story, your purpose, your vision, your possibilities, and your development to consider. The above strategies can only be truly successful after you are considered, first as an individual person.

My main propositions are:

* Just as your body is capable of self-regulation, self-healing, and health maintenance, you are capable of self-development, self-transformation, and authentic life maintenance in such a way as to be able to live a life that is consistent with your purpose, vision, and values;
* A life defined by passion, commitment, and engagement;
* A life of wholeness and presence.
* And just as your body's health sometimes needs some help with its processes, so too does your authentic life need help.

The goal of this book is to provide the first steps of getting you that help. I can't do everything for you – but I can help get you moving in the right direction.

The rest is up to you.

My Story

I was becoming increasingly dissatisfied with my work. Excitement was missing, while there was increasingly dread over the tasks that got in the way of doing the work I wanted to do. I kept pursuing new clinical and non-clinical projects to change things up while trying to still do my already assigned work. I did medical file reviews and question writing for board examination preparation companies. I started workflow projects. I did hospital committee/administration work. I started outpatient clinic sessions in new locations.

Then I woke up and realized that my life was not compatible with my purpose, vision, and values.

Then I figured out WHY and HOW I was sabotaging and limiting myself.

Then I created my map and a navigation system that would bring me to my own authentic physician life.

Then I took action.

(The full version of my story is available on www.drfrancisyoo.com)

Your story

This book's subject matter is you. The content and framework are based on existential philosophy and incorporate elements and ideas from Osteopathic Medicine/Philosophy, Jungian Analytic Psychology and MBTI typology, behavioral economics, the Enneagram, emotional intelligence concepts, and more.

The three parts of this book constitute a step by step guide to realize and actualize your authentic physician life, a life as a physician that is entirely compatible and consistent with your purpose and vision, with what matters to you.

Part I is about waking up and realizing that your life is not compatible with your purpose and vision.

Part II is about learning why and how you sabotage and limit yourself.

Part III is about creating your personalized map and navigation system that will bring you to your own authentic physician life.

By the end, you will be ready to take action with no excuses. You will realize that it is up to you to choose whether or not you will live an engaging, passionate, and committed physician life.

To get there, I am going to challenge you and ask that you challenge yourself.

In fact, here's your first exercise: will you read the rest of this book and see your possibilities for authenticity, or will you stop and return to being stuck in life?

Turn the page if you're ready.

Part I

Your Suffering

Before we do anything else, I want you to congratulate yourself on making the decision to keep turning the page. Welcome to Part I! Here I am going to challenge you to "wake up" to see your current life and how it may be contributing to your suffering. The goal is to bring you to a place of uncomfortable cognitive dissonance.

That's right, the goal is to make you uncomfortable.

Being present with this discomfort offers you a chance to choose and act purposefully in order to move towards your authentic physician life.

Chapter 1

Your Passion

In this chapter you will start this process by defining your vision and mission for your life - and what you are passionate about.

Your vision and mission

Have you ever written your own vision statement and/or mission statement? You may think that "vision statements" and "mission statements" are only for businesses and organizations, but if you were accepted into medical school, you should be answering "Yes." Your personal statement included both your vision and mission and somehow was convincing enough to get you accepted!

So what exactly are your vision and mission?

Your vision is your aspirational, ideal life scenario that you "see" with your inner sense of purpose and authentic self. Your vision statement answers the following (don't answer these yet!):

1) What are you doing in the life that you strive for and aspire to have?

2) Who is involved in what you are doing?

    a. Who are you doing it with? and/or

    b. Who are you doing it for?

Your mission statement consists of all of the assignments or duties to be fulfilled for the sake of the vision. Your mission statement answers the following:

1) How do I achieve my vision?

2) How should I be using my energy, time, and resources to do this?

Please note that you can have multiple missions.

There are plenty of other people who want to tell you how to live your life - what you should strive for and aspire to do as well how to do so. Your parents/guardians, your partner/spouse, your religious organization, the education system, the government, your neighbor next door, the waiter at the restaurant. While they may (or may not) have good intentions, their suggestions may fog up your answers. I am not saying you should not listen to others - you should. However, only <u>you</u> can live your life.

And remember - if you do not figure it out for yourself, it WILL be figured out FOR you.

Example: James Bond is a British secret service agent who is assigned missions to "protect XYZ," "eliminate/capture threat ABC," and others. He completes these missions in order to achieve the ultimate vision, the safety and security of the United Kingdom. Please note that James Bond's vision and mission are already established.

Back to you: Your personal statement said something to the effect of "Your medical school/residency has a mission and vision that is similar to my own and thus getting into, learning at, and graduating from your medical school/residency will help me work on my mission and achieve my vision." In other words, your personal statement conveyed your passion and commitment for your vision and mission and your willingness to engage to make it happen.

Your personal statement

I asked you in the introduction to find your personal statement for medical school and/or residency. You did that, right? If not, go find it now. ...

If you really tried and insist that you cannot find it, that's okay. Try to recall what you wrote then and write it down on paper or type it onto a digital file; do NOT just do the exercise in your mind. It's vital that you actively engage in this step.

Example: Here are a few snippets from my original medical school application statement.

"I believe that the purpose of medicine, of the restoration of health, is to remind people of their own mortality and humanity, and those of others. Intricately related to such a recovery is the rediscovery of the preciousness of life, the rediscovery of the hope they had for certain goals in their lives. With renewed health and re-established hope, people can seek to find projects to work on that will leave positive marks on their lives. The physician's aspiration is to give his/her all in attempting to enable people to realize their goals: to help them to aim towards a project and to be inspired to live life."

"I aim to use medical knowledge to enable people to realize their humanity and to renew their aspirations and hope for achieving significant accomplishments in their lives."

Here is an answer to a specific question for one school I wrote

"Becoming a physician requires a desire for knowledge about the human body and treating it. I believe this would enable me to combine my two great loves: the study of theoretical knowledge, in this case about medicine and the mechanics of the human body, and the putting to practice of a body of knowledge which would be of great direct use, in this case the treating and healing of people."

The vision here is: I am living a life where I work "... to enable people to realize their humanity and to renew their aspirations and hope for achieving significant accomplishment in their lives." The mission is to: Become a physician that learns and applies relevant knowledge to make the vision come true.

Based on my personal statement, it is clear that my commitment to study medicine was driven by a passion for learning and engaging with others' purpose in living. (The word "passion" may bring up various meanings and images for you, which is okay, but please follow along with me. For the purposes of this book, "being passionate" is defined as "having a determined fervor for something.")

Exercise: read through your own personal statement and identify what was the vision and mission there. You may find reading your old writings embarrassing or uncomfortable (I did!); nevertheless, read it. Then, answer the following questions based on your personal statement(s):

- ✓ What were you passionate about? What did you have a fervor and determination for?
- ✓ What did you want to commit yourself to doing?
- ✓ What did you want to fully engage with?

Your current situation

Now consider your current situation. What has changed? Have your vision and mission changed, or are they the same? What are you passionate about, committed to, and desire to engage with now? Have those changed? Take a moment to reflect, but do not answer these now. You are going to answer these questions while writing your new personal statement in Chapter 3, but before we get there, there is something you need to write first in Chapter 2 - your obituary.

Chapter 2

Whose Life Are You Living?

Existential philosophy is concerned with the experience of the individual and how one lives as an individual when faced with one's eventual death and/or one's freedom to choose how to live. Constantly knowing and being keenly aware that your life as you know it will eventually end allows you to contextualize your life and determine whether you are living (or have lived) a meaningful, passionate, authentic life.

Now it is well known that the vague concept of being dead in the future is usually not a great motivator, so we will do an exercise that will help you get into the "existential" mode.

You are going to write your own obituary OR deliver your own eulogy. (Just so that we are on the same page: An obituary is a written description of a recently deceased person's biography published in a newspaper. A eulogy is a verbal account given to honor a deceased person, usually at a funeral. Both the obituary and eulogy typically describe the positive aspects of a person's life.)

Your death and obituary/eulogy

First assume that you will die at about age 80 (unless you are already 80 years of age or older). I realize that your perspective on death will depend on your belief system, and you may do what quantum physicist Hugh Everett III did and ask to be disposed of in the trash after you die. So for the purposes of this book, dying will at the minimum mean to be the cessation of your individual life-sustaining functions in this world.

Second, write your OWN obituary or deliver your OWN eulogy and tell how life will unfold based on how your life is going RIGHT NOW. You can choose one or the other based on your preference for writing or speaking; if you are speaking, I recommend recording it so that you can listen back to it later. Obituaries and eulogies typically focus on the positive aspects of the life of the deceased, but I would like for you to make it as realistic and factual as possible; include the bad with the good.

Here is what a part of mine would look like:

"Dr. Francis Yoo, D.O. went into medicine to apply his medical knowledge to heal and transform people's lives. He spent many, many hours working with patients who did not carry out his recommendations, the reasons for this ranging from flat out refusal to not having the proper resources. He also spent many, many hours learning how to work on inefficient EHR's in order to ensure that the proper CPT codes and modifiers matched up with the necessary ICD-10 codes.

In addition to working as a clinician and battling with the EHR and CPT codes, he took on increasing amounts of work on hospital committees and working on quality improvement projects, was pulled in many directions, and was not able to make and maintain meaningful relationships. He had a variety of interests including existential philosophy and personality type theory but was not able to use them to help his patients because insurance companies would not pay for them."

Your new obituary/eulogy

Third, write another obituary or deliver another eulogy of you, but this time base it on you having lived the life that you dreamed of, one where you accomplished all that you wanted. What have you done? Who were with you? Who did you help? This will end up being a more vivid, flushed out description of your vision in some sense.

Here is what part of mine would look like:

"Dr. Francis Yoo, D.O. went into medicine to apply his medical knowledge to heal and transform people's lives. He started off practicing full-time clinical medicine and doing GME work then transitioned to starting his own businesses where he would have the freedom to focus on and apply his interests in lifestyle medicine, Osteopathy, medical acupuncture, Jungian analytic psychology, the Enneagram, existential philosophy, and more to help people who needed and appreciated his knowledge, expertise, and service without having to worry about insurance companies' interventions, metrics, and restricting EHRs. He was supported by his loving family and like-minded friends and colleagues. He was committed until the day of his death to learn and then teach and utilize his knowledge to engage with others' health and purpose for living."

Every time I read that, I feel inspired – and remember what it is I am aiming for.

Fourth, compare and contrast your two obituaries/eulogies. How similar or different are they? If your two obituaries/eulogies are more or less the same, you probably don't really need to be reading this book!

Your first obituary/eulogy describes your inauthentic life that really is made, or at the very least guided, by others for you to live. It is basically living someone else's life, someone else's vision and mission, and not your own. The second obituary/eulogy describes the authentic life that you consciously chose, pursued, and achieved, a life as a physician filled with passion, commitment, and engagement.

Your discomfort

What reactions did you have at each step of this exercise? You probably felt uncomfortable after Steps #2 and #4. Great!

That was the point. Perhaps you had some sort of negative motion, or your body tensed up, or you rationalized why the two are so different.

This exercise forces you to face your eventual death and deliberate on what really matters to you. Doing the first two steps may have been only somewhat effective in causing some discomfort, but after the final two steps, there should be more of an uncomfortable dissonance because both scenarios came from you so you are MORE motivated to come up with EXCUSES for your current situation and about why this all seems unrealistic or not possible. It brings forth limiting beliefs, inner obstacles, and places that may need to be addressed to move forward, and these are the topics of Part II.

It can be overwhelming at this point to keep going, to keep engaging in the discomfort of your own dissonance, but ask yourself:

Whose life do you want to live?

If your answer is "my own authentic life," then keep reading.

Chapter 3

Face Yourself

Wonderful! You made the decision to turn the page, took action, and turned the page. That means you want to live your own authentic life, right? Then you will have to face yourself.

I had a patient who had oxygen-dependent chronic obstructive pulmonary disease, among other chronic conditions, and who was on multiple medications. The patient had long since stopped tobacco smoking, but the spouse continued to smoke. We counseled the spouse on the detrimental effects smoking would have on both of them multiple times, but it became quickly clear that the spouse had no intention of stopping.

One morning I came into the office and was informed that the patient passed away and that I needed to fill out the death certificate for my patient.

This extreme case illustrates how unchecked inner conflicts and cognitive dissonance can lead to negative outcomes. As with any other person, you have conflicts between motivations, desires, needs, emotions, thoughts, habits, and more. Your decisions and actions are affected by all of these, so in order to be able to make authentic choices, you must face yourself and your inner conflicts.

Your eternal recurrence

The following exercise is based on the *eternal recurrence,* a central aspect of Friedrich Nietzsche's philosophy.

Exercise

Imagine that everything that has ever happened, is happening, and will ever happen will recur again and again an infinite number of times EXACTLY THE SAME WAY EACH TIME. This includes everything from your life - your birth, childhood, what you declared as your undergraduate major(s), which medical schools you applied to and attended, which residency programs you ranked, your career, relationships, death. Would you continue to live the life you are living now knowing that every one of your decisions, experiences, actions you make will repeat an infinite number of times? Your choices and what you do have deep impacts on your life.

Your waking up

In these first three chapters, you explored significant ways that your actions have strayed from your vision, mission, and probably your values. It is easy to shift into some automatic thoughts, feelings, and actions at this juncture - perhaps you rationalized some ifs, whys, and buts, or you started blaming yourself or got angry, or you decided to ignore the whole thing.

However, you cannot choose to change your past nor your decisions and actions up to now.

What you CAN do is choose to acknowledge and accept everything that has led up to now – and then choose to decide where you go next.

Waking up means realizing that your current life may not be aligned with your purpose and vision for your life. Waking up means realizing that you may have in the past and still may be letting others decide your life for you. You have a choice right here, right now:

You can let yourself autopilot away from this inner conflict, or

You can wake up and make a conscious decision to face yourself and your cognitive dissonance.

Your personal statement 2.0

Exercise

Write your new personal statement. You are going to submit this personal statement as part of your "application" to a new training program, a training program made BY you, FOR you. The training program you will explore in Part III will consist of fulfilling your mission by setting goals and objectives, using strategies and tactics, and taking action to reach your vision, your authentic physician life. Use what you've uncovered so far with regards to your inner conflicts between what your life is right now and what you want it to be and map out a new vision/mission for your life.

Once you've finished this new personal statement, continue on to Part II to learn about the many ways you sabotage yourself and how to use that knowledge to increase self-awareness and stay "awake" so that you can work towards making your personal statement 2.0 come true.

Part II

Your Self-sabotage

Welcome to Part II! In Part I, you did the work to identify where your current life is not matching up with your vision and authentic life. Next, you will learn how and why you self-sabotage and, more importantly, how to confront yourself in order to take the next steps towards achieving your vision.

Chapter 4: Why You Self-sabotage

You were born into this world with instincts and reflexes. You reflexively latched on with your mouth to eat as a newborn. You snatched your hand away if you touched something very hot. You instantly become wary around possible dangers, many of which haunt all of us at one time or another: the dark, snakes, being cornered with no way out, heights, loud sounds, or the like.

Instincts for survival (comfort and safety), sexuality (excitement and attraction), and social connection (belonging and contribution) interact with genetic, environmental, and relational factors, and as time goes on, you develop defensive mechanisms and learned behaviors that you apply to protect your ego (defined here as your "daily functioning sense of self").

Your comfortable ego

Your ego craves the comfortable, cozy, and validating nest that your defensive mechanisms and learned behaviors combine to create, and it strategically uses its slew of defenses to protect itself and make sure it stays that safe. This can be helpful or harmful depending on the circumstances.

For example, let's say you grew up with parents or authority figures that rarely, or maybe even never, congratulated you or complimented you when you did your best - you finished eating all of the healthful foods on the plate, you won the watermelon smashing competition, you got an A or 100% on every class and test, you used the $100 you made mowing lawns to make $100,000 by trading options in one year – instead, they always made you feel like you should have done better.

Then your ego will get used to this "not good enough" perspective as being the norm, and everything will be colored by it moving forward. Ordinary daily and extraordinary successes may be followed by feelings of inadequacies or thoughts of how you could have done better, and you may judge yourself to be a failure. Even if you ACTUALLY did a great job and others give you words of accolade, your ego will effectively and efficiently equip itself with honed defenses to stay unmoved and comfortable in this self-defeating posture (more on how the ego does this in Chapter 5).

This is akin to you eating an apple and having a miserable gastroenteritis that makes you very ill with symptoms of fever, malaise, vomiting, and diarrhea and then reacting with disgust or extreme caution when you encounter another apple. The next apple may be a very safe, sanitary apple, but you will still react in such a way to protect yourself as defined by your historical experiences, your learned behaviors, even if it is logically clear to you (and anyone watching) that it should be fine to eat the apple.

Your sympathetic nervous system

Imagine the following scenarios:

> ➢ You are in a pool for the first time in ages, and you notice a hungry shark raise its head above the pool water.

- ➤ You are giving a presentation at a national conference that you have never been to before with a room full of strangers, and you notice several people yawning or laughing as you talk.
- ➤ You are driving down a dark, foggy road when a deer jumps out of the bushes and onto the road in front of you.
- ➤ You get a letter claiming to be from the IRS stating "Open immediately upon receipt!"

In each of those moments, your sympathetic nervous system prepares you to fight, fly, or freeze. You sweat and feel warm, your hands tremble, your heart and respiratory rates increase. You feel afraid and alert. Your thoughts either accelerate or stop.

I hope you agree that crashing into a deer or being attacked by a shark can be deadly, and that having such a reaction makes sense. However, you will not actually die from speaking publicly where everyone's attention is on you or if you get a letter claiming to be from a government organization with a warning.

But you very well may feel like you might die. Your *entire being* is involved in any fear reaction, regardless of the source.

Your psyche may become sensitized and upregulated in a similar way so that the nervous system becomes sensitized to perceived increased pain, even with less or no nociceptive input. You may avoid pools, public speaking, driving, or looking at the mail at all because of the ego's attempt to be ready "just in case," arising from an understandable desire to avoid what feel like deadly situations.

This is not bad in itself if the threat to your safety or life is high enough.

However it IS detrimental if you get these reactions while performing every day, non-deadly tasks. This is extremely important to keep in mind when you are faced with the chance to make decisions and perform actions that you have not done before but that will be ultimately beneficial - the ego would like you to say "no" to such decisions and actions so you can be cozy and comfortable, but that is not necessarily what will get you to your authentic life.

Your status quo

Your sympathetic nervous system and ego have really good intentions - to make sure you're alive and able to deal with everyday life! On the other hand, when the autonomic nervous system becomes unbalanced and leans toward hyperactivity of the sympathetic nervous system, it is ultimately harmful. Similarly, if your psyche becomes unbalanced and tilts towards the ego hyperactively trying to safeguard a comfortable image of itself, the psyche sees the steps required to live an authentic life as being risky. Your ego perceives your desire to live a balanced and authentic, purposeful life in pursuit of your vision to be a threat to the not-so-great, suboptimal yet functioning status quo.

THIS is a major reason why you self-sabotage: because your ego tries to play it safe to keep you safe in the short-term, even if that keeps you from achieving your vision in the long-term.

Now that you know why you self-sabotage, you will learn in Chapter 5 the various strategies and tactics your ego uses to interrupt your desire for authentic living - that is, how you self-sabotage.

Chapter 5

How You Self-sabotage: Part 1

In the last chapter, you learned why you self-sabotage when you try to seek your authentic life: your ego structures a comfortable, cozy, internally-valid status quo that sees attempts to transform and grow as threatening and risky. In this chapter, you will learn the strategies and some of the tactics that the ego uses.

Your ego's strategy

Your ego essentially wants to maintain the status quo of its self-image. It constructs a web of automatic physiological, emotional, cognitive, and behavioral reactions. It then coaxes you into the comfort and coziness of this web while trying to make you forget that you are actually stuck and trapped by the web!

Your ego wants you to fall asleep to your authenticity and live life satisfied with the way it is going.

Now this does not mean the ego does not want anything to change. The ego wants decisions and actions, whether major and dramatic or minor and miniscule, that will ultimately maintain the status quo of self-image of the ego. For example, a physician may choose a specialty, a spouse, a house, or even a car, all mainly to reinforce the self-image of feeling important, wealthy, and successful.

Your ego's tactics

Your ego's tactics consist of the following: psychological defense mechanisms; cognitive biases; automatic physiological, emotional, cognitive, and/or behavioral reactions; and distortions in our thinking, feeling, doing. Again, here's a reminder - these things can be protective and are not bad, per se, but they can become limiting and ultimately are not conducive to authenticity and personal development.

Your defense mechanisms

Defense mechanisms are ways that the mind deals with information in order to diffuse anxiety and impulses in such a way as to maintain one's worldview (or more specifically, the ego's status quo). Examples of defense mechanisms include:

Denial: You experience worsening symptoms that probably indicate a pathological process that needs medical attention but refuse the possibility that you are sick and instead continue to live life and go to work as if nothing is wrong.

Projection: You harbor anger at the deli employee for taking too long to make your breakfast sandwich, an action that could make you late, but really you're late because *you* snoozed too many times that morning.

Repression: You block out the memory of your patient who died during a prolonged and highly emotional code that you were leading.

Rationalization: You are treated badly by a boss/attending and rationalize that it's okay since "it's just how it is around here, and I'm used to it now."

Withdrawal/Avoidance: If you are not looking forward to being dead, you avoid thinking about it.

Humor: You feel awkward while on a long, cramped elevator ride with another person and make a joke.

Your cognitive biases

Cognitive biases are systematic structures and patterns that the mind employs to make decisions more easily at the expense of objectivity. Cognitive biases are not good or bad in themselves *per se* because they function as mental shortcuts to make living easier.

Here are some examples:

Confirmation bias: You do an online search of the number of physicians who are dissatisfied with their current career and focus only on the ones that confirm/agree with your viewpoint and dismiss, ignore, or downplay the ones that do not. That is, you look and "see" only the sources that confirm your stance.

Escalation of commitment: You realize years into your clinical career that you absolutely hate the specialty but do not look for other options and continue with the same job at the same location because you think it is "too late to change."

Planning fallacy and optimism bias: You are working full-time at your current job and decide to increase your hours for additional income, believing it will work out fine because you somehow made it work at your previous workplace. "I made it work before, so it will work out this time too."

Curse of knowledge: You start discussing the pros and cons of doing clinical medicine full-time versus part-time to first year undergraduate pre-med students who have never been employed before.

IKEA effect: You make a website (first time ever!) for your practice and you know it has a lot room for improvement, but you think it is absolutely as remarkable and good as the websites of other practices made by professional designers.

(Recommendation: *Thinking, Fast and Slow* by Daniel Kahneman, Ph.D and winner of the 2002 Nobel Memorial Prize in Economic Sciences. It is a great (but long) book to learn about many cognitive biases. His is a behavioral economics perspective, but the concepts can easily be used in different settings.)

Your self-awareness

Your self-defense mechanisms and cognitive biases are powerful tactics used by your ego to protect the status quo and let you function more efficiently throughout the day, but that protection and function come at the expense of potential self-awareness, personal development and transformation, and a chance to be conscious of your ability to choose and realize your vision of your authentic physician life. Knowing when, why, and how to use certain defense mechanisms and cognitive biases is essential for staying awake and to remain focused on living life towards your vision.

(Go to www.drfrancisyoo.com for more discussions about defense mechanisms and cognitive biases and additional tools for self-awareness).

Chapter 6

How You Self-sabotage: Part 2

Continuing on with Part II's theme of learning to be aware of how self-sabotage prevents you from living your authentic physician life, you will learn in this chapter about how you self-sabotage based on concepts from the Myers-Briggs Type Indicator (MBTI) typology/Jungian Analytic Psychology and Enneagram.

Your MBTI Type

The MBTI is a set of questions that is designed to help you find your "personality" type out of 16 possible ones and is derived from psychiatrist Dr. Carl Gustav Jung, M.D.'s typology system. It takes into account your natural preferences on receiving information and making decisions. Each of the 16 types has their own strengths, weakness, opportunities, and threats.

I recently posted this question in various physician Facebook groups:

"Has anyone here used the Myers-Briggs Type Indicator (MBTI) and/or Jungian typology for personal development on a level past "taking an online questionnaire" and a casual understanding?"

While I was interested in the diversity of answers as a certified MBTI practitioner, I was more amazed at the vitriolic answers provided by otherwise well-educated physicians whose knowledge about the subject was mostly misconceptions and falsehoods (a striking illustration of a Dunning–Kruger effect cognitive bias).

Knowing your best-fit MBTI type and/or the various cognitive functions associated with the same are helpful in identifying your behavior patterns as well as how you sabotage yourself. For example, my MBTI type has the propensity to be imaginative and come up with new ideas but has a harder time with sensory input. For example, I have to drive the same route with the same starting point and destination more than twenty times with the help of a GPS before I can do the same drive without it.

On the other hand, people with other MBTI types may over-rely on established methods and disregard innovative ideas until they become more "mainstream" (new medical treatments are a great example). You can see how gaining insight into some of the preferences that you manifest and depend upon all the time could be helpful in getting you to wake up and get out of your ego's cruise control.

A few warnings about misconceptions about the MBTI: I implore you, please do not answer questions you find on a random website and think the end result is your type. Not only is this the wrong way to do it, it can be potentially harmful to your self-awareness. Also, the MBTI is NOT a "test;" it is not something you can pass or fail. If you are interested in how to do it the right way, e-mail me or go to my website at www.drfrancisyoo.com (I am certified by the Center of Applications of Psychological Type: https://www.capt.org).

Your Enneagram Type

The Enneagram (literally nine-written/drawn) is a nine-pointed figure that is the symbol used in the system named after this figure. It is increasingly being used as a sort of personality typology system whose nine main types are distinguished by key underlying motivations and patterns of distortions in thoughts, emotions, and actions. As someone who has taken over two hundred hours of training at the Enneagram Institute, I recommend the RHETI (a not-free indicator; at www.enneagraminstitute.com/rheti) and David Daniels' process in his book "Essential Enneagram: The Definitive Personality Test and Self-Discovery Guide"

My concept of "waking up" comes from my Enneagram education, and indeed it is a great system that if applied correctly can help you identify the automatic reactions and distortions in your thoughts, emotions, and actions.

Distortions and automatic reactions

I explained earlier about how your ego does a lot to maintain a cruise control or status quo of your self-image, even if it may be potentially harmful or damaging in some ways. The Enneagram describes how each of the nine types goes into "cruise control" and their associated distortions.

For example, based on my Enneagram type, being in unfamiliar situations triggers my ego's desire for the status quo and causes the automatic thought, "I don't know what I'm doing," automatic feeling of anxiety, and the automatic impulse to withdraw from others and into my thoughts, as well as try to become competent by attending a multitude of courses and reading many books. However, this is a distortion of reality as I am knowledgeable now and have been able to successfully apply what I learned.

Your responsibility

I do not intend to go through all of the MBTI and Enneagram types and the many nuances therein, but I hope you get an idea how they have helped me and can help you see how your defense mechanisms, cognitive biases, automatic patterned thoughts/ emotions/behaviors, and distortions can interfere with defining and pursuing your vision for your life.

The more insight you gain from knowing your MBTI and Enneagram type, the more helpful it will be in identifying your self-sabotaging patterns.

Think about how many of your choices were driven by defense mechanisms, cognitive biases, automatic reactions, and distortions as opposed to being made from a state of self-awareness. Acquiring the essential insight into the ways that you self-sabotage can be immensely helpful in helping you to be responsible by giving you a better chance to actually RESPOND from a more aware state instead of REACTING from the ego's desire for status quo maintenance.

Now that you have a good sense of why and how you sabotage yourself, we can transition to Part III where you will pick up some practical insights and tools that will allow you to move ever closer to living your authentic physician life.

Part III

Your Map and Navigation System

In Part I, you were asked to wake up and truly face yourself, mainly by having you contrast aspects of your current life with the authentic physician life that is truly aligned with your vision. In Part II, you were introduced to the why and how of your self-sabotage. In Part III, you will determine your definitive purpose and plan that connect the profound depths of your being with practical steps you can start to take today.

Chapter 7

Your Definitive Purpose and Plan: Part 1

Having a map and a navigation system make traveling much easier, especially if you are going to a location you have not been to before. Along these lines, adequate preparation before any journey is essential, but note that it is possible to over-prepare, which leads to lack of taking action. This procrastination, whether purposeful or not, is quite inefficient. Keep this in mind as take a look at one representation of the map that we've developed to get you where you need to go.

First, take a look at this awesome drawing:

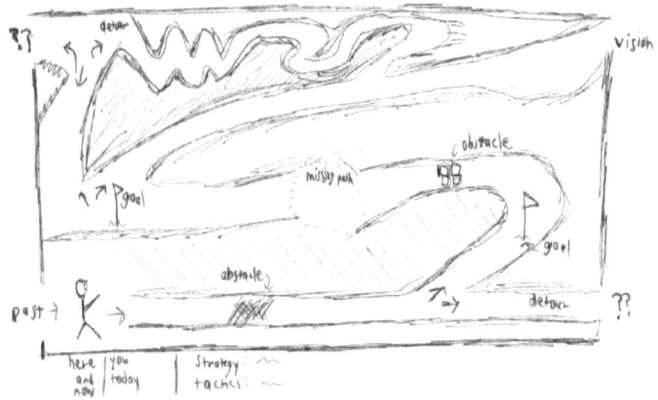

Here is the legend

Origin = starting point

Vision = the destination

Mission = the overall layout of the intended path you are to journey on

Goal = landmarks that are clear markers of getting closer to the destination

Objective = the coordinates of the landmarks

Obstacles blocking the path

Missing areas on the path

Detours = diversions or deviations from your intended path

Strategy = how to stay on this path

Tactic = how to get to the next step

Action steps = each step on the path

Your starting point

Your starting point is a thorough description of yourself and your "inventory." "Yourself" refers to internal aspects, while "your inventory" refers to external aspects.

Yourself:

- ✓ Physical qualities: body measurements and characteristics, physical health
- ✓ Other quantitative measures: age, location, genetic/heritage background, upbringing
- ✓ Inborn (or untaught) qualities: abilities, intuition, interests
- ✓ Gained qualities: skills, knowledge, degrees, credentials
- ✓ Habits including cognitive biases, defense mechanisms, emotional reactions, behavior
- ✓ What you spend your money and time on

- ✓ Your values, purpose, vision, calling
- ✓ Attitude towards your environment and the natural world (earth, nature)

Your beliefs:
- ✓ Religious
- ✓ Spiritual
- ✓ Philosophical
- ✓ Ethical
- ✓ Worldview

Your inventory:
- ✓ Possessions
- ✓ Physical possessions
- ✓ Financials: assets and liabilities, sources of income
- ✓ Insurance products: disability, life, home, car, umbrella, etc.
- ✓ Living situation
- ✓ Relationships
- ✓ Relationships with specific people
- ✓ Innermost circle of family, friends, colleagues, community, pets

- ✓ Still close but not quite innermost people
- ✓ Mentors, teachers, etc
- ✓ Everyone else you know
- ✓ Everyone you don't know
- ✓ Relationships with groups of people
- ✓ Organizations, nations, parties

Note that I did not include "time" here. It is not part of your inventory because you cannot control time. (Unless you know something I don't. If so, let me know!)

Exercise

Write down the aspects about "yourself" and your "inventory" based on the above list. You can also think of it as a "CV for your life." Feel free to add to it. It may take some time to do this. You will need this information for chapters 8 and 9, so please complete the list either now before moving on or after reading the whole book when you come back to do the exercises.

Your destination (vision)

I am going to be using the terms "vision" and "mission" in a particular way once again, so I will define them here to be absolutely certain we are on the same page. Have your second obituary/eulogy and personal statement 2.0 available.

Your vision is the aspirational ideal that you vividly depicted in your second obituary. It describes the following

What are you doing? What does your typical day or week look like?

Who are you with? Who are you surrounded by or who are you interacting with?

What change are you making? Who are you helping, directly or indirectly? How is the world being changed?

Your path (mission)

Your mission is that which needs to be happening to reach your vision. Think of it as being dispatched on an assignment to fulfill a duty... the duty that brings your reality closer to your vision. Your mission continually brings you closer to and supports your vision.

Exercise

Use your second obituary/eulogy and personal statement 2.0 as guidelines to flush out your vision and mission. You may get some new ideas while you do this. This part is important.

Let me be clear as to how important.

There is <u>no</u> point in reading this book if you do not do this. You can check out mine at www.drfrancisyoo.com if you need some inspiration.

Ok, you're done with writing out your vision and mission. Good!

Take a look again at the map. Your vision is the destination on your map, and your mission is the path that will bring you to your destination.

Chapter 8

Your Definitive Purpose and Plan: Part 2

Take a good look at the path (mission) that will take you to your destination (vision). You will see three different kinds of objects as well as paths diverging from the main path. These three objects are:

Landmarks = goals and objectives

Obstacles = prevent you from moving forward by blocking the path forward.

Missing roads = prevent you from moving forward by the absence of a road to take.

Your landmarks

Goals are the results you need to achieve in order to complete the mission, while your objectives are measurable targets that help determine if you have accomplished your goals. On the map, your goals are landmarks or sites where you can put up a flag when you get there. They can act as signs of having accomplished something and gotten closer to your destination.

Your objectives are the coordinates of your goals. How will you know you reached the correct landmark if you don't know its specific location? For example, "pay off my medical student loan debt" is a goal while "have $0 in student loan debt within five years after completing residency" is an objective.

Your obstacles

Your obstacles are aspects about yourself or inventory that need to be decreased, removed, or changed in some way. The starting point to identify your obstacles is to take a look at how you sabotage yourself. (Nearly) all of your obstacles originate from the defense mechanisms, cognitive biases, and automatic reactions and distortions that you learned about in Part II.

Let's use the example of starting your own cash-only, private clinical practice as the goal for here and the rest of this chapter.

Examples:

Defense mechanism - delaying the work needed to learn about what is required to start a practice by watching shows on Netflix because it just seems overwhelming to start.

Automatic reaction - thinking and believing "I will not succeed, so why start?" which is accompanied by anxiety.

Cognitive bias/confirmation bias - reading that more and more physicians are transitioning to being employed while ignoring news about physicians starting new private practices.

The key point here is that you will not even realize these obstacles are there if you are not aware of them or looking for them.

Your missing roads

Your missing roads are aspects of yourself or inventory that are lacking and need to be increased, gained, or positively changed in some way. A good starting point for identifying the missing roads is taking a look at some of the aspects of yourself you wrote down in Chapter 7.

Examples:

Lack of knowledge - learning the legal and/or financial needs to start a practice

Lack of funds - not having the money to pay for legal and other fees

Lack of a practice location – not having a physical location to see patients at

Your detours

Besides your starting point, destination, path to the destination, landmarks, obstacles, and missing roads, there are also paths that diverge from the path to the destination. These detours are diversions or deviations from your intended path. They may either slow you down or take you in a completely different direction!

Examples:

Pursuing an MBA degree so that you can start a business/practice

Continuing to work full-time as an employee in a job you do not like and that does not allow you to give intention and attention to starting your practice

Figuring out the intricacies of how insurance companies reimburse physicians for the services you want to give in your practice

I to emphasize here that you cannot change what happened in the past so do not call anything you did in the past a detour. Everything you did in the past is now a part of you and your inventory.

Exercise

Start a list of your goals and related objectives, obstacles, missing roads, and detours. It does not need to be perfect. Just get it started with at least a few items on each. If you are not sure about where one would go, put it under a "sort later" category.

Now that you have your map, go on to Chapter 9 where you will learn how to start putting your navigation system together.

Chapter 9

Your Navigation System

In Chapters 7 and 8, you learned how to draw your own map for authentic physician living. It is now time to create your navigation system: your strategy and tactics. Your strategy is how you will conduct, carry out, and complete the mission. It is the master plan that you will use to proceed past obstacles, missing roads, and detours on your path (mission) to your destination (vision). Your tactics are the techniques, vehicles, and tools to use to deal with specific obstacles, missing roads, and detours.

Think of your strategy as the operating system of your navigation system on your smartphone or automobile computer and the tactics are what need to be loaded onto your operating system so that you can actually use your navigation system.

Your general strategy has two components: self-management and task-management. Here are a few immediately useful tactics for each of these.

Your self-management

Self-management is a strategy that involves self-awareness, inner work, and personal development with the aim of improving the ability to identify, process, and respond to stressors and their effect on you. This involves ways to deal with your defense mechanisms, cognitive biases, automatic reactions, and distortions. This includes what people often term "changing your mindset" and attitude.

Self-management tactics include: cognitive behavior therapy techniques, modeling the behavior of someone who is successful, meditative introspective practices, prayer, getting the help or advice of others, image-training (visualizing your realized goal or vision), self-reminders (put up post-it note reminders to remind and motivate you about your vision or any other aspect of your map), developing a habit by doing it every day for a given time frame (3 months). Another good one is spending time around people who are positive, inspirational, and otherwise elevate and motivate you to move forward.

If you have been doing all of my exercises, you have already started to use some of my favorite self-management tactics. Identifying how you sabotage yourself gives you insight into your strengths, weaknesses, opportunities, and threats. Learning and studying your MBTI type and functions and Enneagram type are also self-management tactics.

Your task management

Task management is choosing which tasks to address with your intention and attention. In other words, it is prioritizing your tasks. You have full freedom, control, and choice over which tasks you decide to be involved in.

One great tactic you can start using right away is the "task sorter." Here's how it works:

1) List the tasks that are being done right now, i.e. your current state of affairs. 2) Identify which of these tasks are detours and which ones bring you closer to your next goal.

2) Put the un-needed tasks (detours) on your "not-to-do" list.

3) List the tasks that need to be done.

4) Identify which ones can be done by someone else. Put these on the "someone else to do" list.

5) Everything else goes on your "to do list"

You should now have the following lists:

> Not-to-do list - Dispose of these tasks.

> Someone-else-to-do list - Delegate these tasks to other people.

> To-do-list - You should only be focusing on these tasks.

Let's go back to the example of starting your own cash-only clinical practice. It is ultimately up to you which tasks get put on which list depending on your map, but this should give you an idea of what that might look like:

Not-to-do list - Negotiate with insurance companies, get an MBA degree.

Someone-else-to-do list - Design and maintain your practice website, answer phone calls and make appointments, take vital signs of patients.

To-do-list - Care for patients, find people to help you.

Your help

Acknowledge and accept this phrase: "I need help." Say it out loud. Let it be known to yourself and to others. It is tempting to do everything yourself. I should know. I've been there. You need help. And I do not mean your family member or friend that happens to be the closest person to you right now. I mean the *actual* people that can *actually* help you with what you *actually* need.

Examples of help:

Mentor - Someone who has already succeeded in what you are trying to do.

Coach - Someone who provides training and guidance that you need and keeps you accountable.

Consultant - Someone who specializes in fixing a specific problem, e.g., starting a cash private-practice.

Physician/healer - Let's face it: you may need a physician or healer of some sort.

Financial advisor - Many physicians would rather have someone help manage their investments.

Lawyer, accountant, religious/spiritual leader, representative from a medical organization.

Besides getting the help of specific people, you need to gain knowledge either from books, courses (online or in person), formal education, or somewhere/someone else. Which resources you need is entirely dependent on your needs.

And when you are not sure what resources you need, just start somewhere and ask for help.

Conclusion

Your Authentic Physician Life

In Part I, you woke up to the discrepancy between your current life and your vision for your authentic physician life.

In Part II, you learned about why and how you sabotage yourself from taking action to get closer to your vision.

In Part III, you made your personal map and navigation system that constitute your definitive purpose and plan for your authentic physician life.

It is now time to put all of this together.

Your next step

Review your list of obstacles, missing roads, and detours. Which of them is the "key lesion?" By this I mean, which of these is the one thing that if you address it, everything else will start to fall into place or become easier to accomplish? Your immediate next step is to identify what YOU need to do to overcome that key lesion and which one of your tactics (tools, techniques, vehicles) you need to utilize to do so.

Maybe it is to ask colleagues for recommendations for a CPA, to attend the conference on non-clinical careers for physicians given by XYZ annually in October, choosing which of the services in your clinical practice you need to focus on and which ones to stop, taking time to engage in serious introspection, rereading this book and doing all of the exercises, or finding a mentor.

Once you decide on a specific task, you can make that action step/task into a "sub-goal" and then figure out that goal's objectives, needed strategy and tactics, and action steps.

For example: You decide that your task and sub-goal is to find a mentor that will help you start your cash-only private practice. Your objective is to find a physician who has started the type of practice you want to run within one month and have them help you. Your strategy might center on searching for possible candidates and influencing them to help you. Your tactics for influence could be some of the tools to connect with others as suggested in Keith Ferrazzi's book "Never Eat Alone." This is just one way your next step might look. Your actual step would depend on what you figured out so far by doing the exercises in this book.

You have no excuses

If you completed all the exercises, you should have a clear idea of the tasks you need to accomplish next. You know which tactics you need to perform those tasks. These are specific parts of your strategy (master plan) to accomplish your goals (landmarks) in order to work on your overall mission (intended path) to eventually reach your vision (destination).

This means that everything on your map and navigation system are coherent and in consonance. You can trace everything from your vision to your next action; you can trace your action steps all the way to your vision and see how they are connected because it was all created from your authentic self.

What this really means is that you have no excuses.

Absolutely, NO excuses.

(Note that you will update aspects of your map and navigation system as you go down your path (mission) as you learn new things and changes happen during your journey. This is normal – don't let it deter or detour you.)

Your decision

You faced the dissonance between your current reality and how you really want to live life and came face to face with your authentic physician life.

You faced your self-sabotaging methods.

You faced your authentic map for a definitive purpose and plan.

But before you go do anything, before you CAN do anything else, there is one thing you must do first:

You must face yourself and your fate to be free to choose.

With great freedom comes great responsibility,

And you must decide.

Not deciding means letting someone else decide for you.

Will you choose to be committed to your mission and vision?

Or will you choose to betray yourself?

Will you choose to passionately engage with life?

Or will you drift away from yourself?

Will you choose to become who you really care to be?

Or will you become someone else?

Will you choose to be authentic?

Or will you live someone else's life?

Will you choose to live your authentic physician life?

Post-script: Q&A

Here is a Q&A for common questions or retorts that I anticipate.

This sounds great and all... but it is just not practical.

It cannot NOT be practical because you are the one that makes your own map and navigation system. The tricky part is that our self-sabotage system functions so well that it is usually difficult to see all aspects of ourselves. I advise you to go over your vision and mission again and this time try to see what defense mechanisms, cognitive biases, automatic reactions, and distortions come up. Get help with this if needed.

What if someone's vision or mission is nefarious or is otherwise harmful to others?

Each person's map and navigation system is regulated and balanced internally. In most cases, if the reader truly considers their defense mechanisms, cognitive biases, automatic reactions, and distortions, they will understand that they need to get help figuring out those difficulties and any derangements they have in their vision and mission

I did all of the exercises but am having trouble taking the first step and making my decision. What should I do?

What is really holding you back is inside you and nowhere else. What are you afraid of?

Acknowledge and accept you need help. Whose help do you need?

Where can I learn more about XYZ?

I did indeed condense a lot of information into this book. I wrote this book in a way that would trigger you and get you started. You can start by joining my Facebook group "Physician Freedom: Living Your Authentic Physician Life":

www.facebook.com/groups/AuthenticPhysicianLife

Also, check out my website at www.drfrancisyoo.com. Or you can e-mail me at dr.francisyoo@gmail.com, if there is something in this book that you want more information about.

Isn't this way of thinking and deciding selfish?

Yes, I suppose it can be seen that way. I believe that if everyone is living authentic lives where they can fully engage with whatever they are committed to doing, everyone would be happier, more productive, and more able to help themselves, each other, and the world. The reason that there are so many people unhappy with their work is because they convince themselves they have no other choice and force themselves into a position that is probably a better fit for someone else. Also, it is not your job to fix every single thing and have a solution for every problem. So yes, living your authentic physician life will benefit you, but ultimately your loved ones and the whole world.

This all sounds great, but I am still stuck.

This book's content was meant to get you started. If you need more help, you can start by joining my Facebook group "Physician Freedom: Living Your Authentic Physician Life," check out my website www.drfrancisyoo.com. Or e-mail me here:

dr.francisyoo@gmail.com.

What do you mean by "self?"

The main issue with discussing what the "self" means is that the word is used to mean many things in various psychological, philosophical, and religious schools of thought as well as in more everyday usage. For the purposes of this book, I use the word "self" to indicate the observable and discernable aspects of a person.

Questions, comments, etc?

Again, consider joining my Facebook group "Physician Freedom: Living Your Authentic Physician Life":

www.facebook.com/groups/AuthenticPhysicianLife

Check out my website, www.drfrancisyoo.com, where I will address further questions, or emailing me at dr.francisyoo@gmail.com.

Acknowledgments

First, I want to generally acknowledge my mentors, family, and friends, and everyone who put up with me... and continues to do so.

More specific gratitude to:

My mother 유 중희 and father 유 원국

FUMC KYG/YG & ssn's

Suite 607/Chili Dog Night

The (left) back row academic caucus

RPSOM

Atlus

Gust

KyoAni

Nintendo

Square-Enix

Dr. Lawrence Barnard, DO

Dr. Charles Beck, DO

Dr. Shawn Cannon, DO

Dr. Lauren Davis, DO

Dr. Richard Feely, DO

Philip Gwak

Dr. Donald Hankinson, DO

支倉 凍砂 (Isuna Hasekura)

Russ Hudson

梶浦 由記 (Yuki Kajiura)

Julian Kim

Dr. Carl Gustav Jung, MD

Søren Aabye Kierkegaard

Tara Lavery

Dr. Christopher Loo, MD, PhD

光田 康典 (Yasunori Mitsuda)

Karen Roberts

坂口 博信 (Hironobu Sakaguchi)

Professor Robert C. Solomon, PhD

高橋 哲哉 (Tetsuya Takahashi)

橙乃 ままれ (Mamare Touno)

植松 伸夫 (Nobuo Uematsu)

Dr. Daniel VanArsdale, DO
Dr. Craig Wells, DO
Dr. Mike Woo-Ming, MD
Dr. Sheldon Yao, DO
Ἰησοῦ Χριστοῦ

About the Author

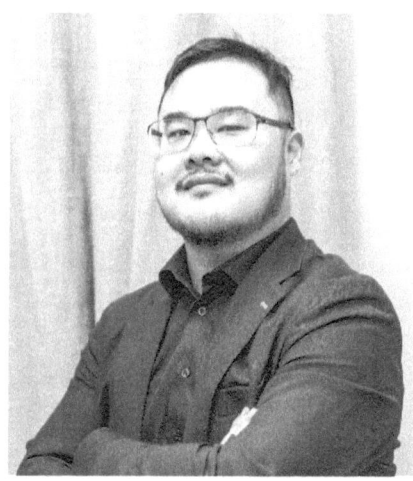

So you want to know about Francis Yoo? He's an interesting guy.

Or at least he thinks he is.

He is a perennial nerd.

He attended and graduated from Hunter College High School. Then he earned his B.A. in Mathematics and Philosophy in the College of Arts and Sciences at New York University while fulfilling pre-med requirements. Next up was a Doctor of Osteopathic Medicine degree from the New York College of Osteopathic Medicine. He did his post-graduate training at Southampton Hospital.

He is certified by the American Osteopathic Board of Family Practice, the American Osteopathic Board of Neuromusculoskeletal Medicine, ABPS in Integrative Medicine, and possesses additional qualification in Pain Medicine by the American Osteopathic Association. He is a Diplomate of the American Board of Medical Acupuncture and the Center for Education and Development in Homeopathy.

He is also a certified MBTI practitioner (CAPT/CPP). He is a Lean Six Sigma green belt and has completed the Riso Hudson Certified Enneagram Teacher Curriculum.

So, what does he do with all of this? One of his biggest interests is integrating it all to create practical authentically life-transforming applications to help others, especially physicians that having difficulty making career decisions. Another one is integrating Osteopathy, Jungian Analytic Psychology, and the

Enneagram for body-mind-spirit medicine, health, well-being, and development.

Now only if he can find a way to incorporate music creation into all of this, too! His weapon of choice is the electric guitar with a lot of distortion.

He also loves sushi and pizza... just not at the same time.

He always wanted to write and publish a book (he has that covered now).

He serves as a deacon at the First United Methodist Church in Flushing.

He unapologetically loves JRPGs.

He wishes he could be really good at the Touhou Project games.

His website is www.drfrancisyoo.com

His e-mail address is dr.francisyoo@gmail.com

Check out the companion Facebook group to this book, "Physician Freedom: Living Your Authentic Physician Life."